Searching for Cecy:
Reflections on Alzheimer's

Judy Prescott

First published by
Live Consciously Publishing in 2012.
Printed and bound in the United States.

ISBN: 978-0-9554656-1-1

Library of Congress Cataloging-in-Publication Data on file.
Control Number: 2011931817

Cover and interior design by David San Miguel
Art photography by Alisa Copenhaver
Cover art by Anne Gresinger © 2012
Typefaces: Stempel Schneidler Std, Garamond LT Std

Live Consciously Publishing
665 Walther Way
Los Angeles, CA 90049

www.liveconsciouslynow.com

For my brothers

"We make out of the quarrel with others, rhetoric,
but of the quarrel with ourselves, poetry."
—W.B. Yeats

Contents

Introduction   *viii*

Acknowledgments   *x*

THE FOG   **I.**

2   Painted Wings

4   Measuring Up

6   The Seagull

8   Mother's Lullaby

NOR'EASTER   **II.**

12   Proof

14   Gone

16   Quick Hold

18   Mother

EBB TIDE   **III.**

22   Silent Sea

24   Unveiled

26   Vanishing

28   Home

30   Firefly

MACKEREL SKY   **IV.**

34   Sexy and Cecy

36   Fishing Nets

IN IRONS   V.

40 Motherless Mom

42 Bon Voyage

FOLLOWING SEA   VI.

46 "Let's Just Get Home,"
    she said…

48 Fledglings

50 Hello

52 Safe Passage

54 Birds of a Feather

RED, RIGHT, RETURNING   VII.

58 Seizures

60 Irony Lost

62 Mirage

64 In Confidence

66 I Hear You

68 Stymied

70 Resolute

Introduction

I had to take a sudden tack in 1999 when my mother, Mary Boodell Prescott, a.k.a. "Cecy," began exhibiting signs of early-onset Alzheimer's disease. I learned, under the guidance of those who navigate Cecy's world daily, how best to chart my course. Cecy moves the extraordinary people who care for her in the same way she moved those of us who knew her before her transformation. These kind, unsung heroes help my mother to feel safe and valued. I am forever in their debt. They divine beauty from chaos, order from confusion and have become her home.

I have learned to quietly step into Cecy's world, leaving all of our shared history behind me. Every moment with my mother is entirely new...there is no before or after. She remains a scintillating, funny woman who is a pleasure to spend time with.

I began writing poetry at the age of thirteen when my closest childhood friend, Kyle, died of heart failure. I was quickly advised to hide my feelings in the event that my tears might further upset her already grief-stricken family. Swallowing hard and facing a completely new reality, I turned to my pen. This was the beginning of a habit for me...a new way of coping. I write to understand.

My mother took a great interest in my poetry and helped me to edit my work. An English major who could do the Sunday New York Times crossword puzzle in an hour, she was no slouch with words. She often asked why I never wrote about her. I told her to be careful what she wished for and ironically, she won out in the end.

These poems span an eight-year period. The first few were written when Cecy was still living in her home and in great need of help. Those that follow reflect her transition to assisted living and finally to the Alzheimer's facility where she lives today. The poems are arranged chronologically and are matched with artwork contributed by family artists in honor of my mother. These beautiful pieces deepen my work and help to track both my emotional journey and the progression of a disease.

This work represents my best effort to understand and celebrate the remarkable woman who introduced me to her great loves: Renata Tebaldi, Gelsey Kirkland, Graham Greene, E.E. Cummings, John Wayne and the Chicago Bears. I felt a need to reflect on the life of the reluctant debutante who could play Chopin flawlessly, dance the Carolina Shag with wild abandon, and throw up a spinnaker in record time. She is a class act and I miss her. She is simply Cecy, the same as she ever was…a beautiful soul that wishes to be heard… a rare, complicated person whom I am proud to call "Mom."

This is my tribute to her.

Acknowledgments

Many thanks to the four Maine artists whose work graces the pages of this book. Cecy is so fond of Maine and would be honored to know that these four relatives have contributed their talent and insight to celebrate her: Tom Prescott, Rosanne Prescott MacPherson, Anne Gresinger, and Susan Winn. Thank you.

I am very grateful to my uncle, Tom Boodell, for his fine example and for reminding me that there is decency and justice in the world. His love of letters and his continued quest for knowledge inspire me. It was he who gave Mom the nickname "Cecy" as a child because he couldn't say "sister." Uncle Tom's daughter, Mary, has been a continual source of strength for me throughout this great struggle. She loves my mother, her godmother, as I do, and for that love, I am eternally grateful.

I thank my brothers, Tom and John, for their will to keep us together after the battering winds of Alzheimer's attempted to blow us apart. We are all indebted to Tom for his constant care of Cecy. I am also beholden to my brother John, Eliza's godfather, who told me, when I was expecting, that regardless of his low voice, he could be the mother I needed. Thanks also, to our father, Don Prescott, for frequently visiting Mom when we needed his support.

I give heartfelt appreciation to Cecy's kind friends who have stepped in for me when she needed to step out: Dee Benson, Beata Boodell, Sandi Boynton, Sherry Corbett, Lee Dursin, Martie Harrigan, Ginny Irwin, Rosanne MacPherson, Danne Munford, Mary Pelikan, Jean Rizzo, Monica Shirvanian, and Nadeshiko Yamaguchi. My journey has been easier because of you.

Thank you to the staff of Hawthorne House for their devotion to Cecy and to Nancy Thayer who regularly looks in on Mom when I am so far away. A special thanks to Linda Brown and Corinne Lanpher for their continued devotion to Cecy even though she is no longer in their care, and to David Shaul for his shared experience and constant encouragement.

Humble thanks to my editor and childhood friend, Cindy Jeck Davis, for her fine mind and exquisite insight and to Eileen Gibson Funke for her keen eye and for putting me in the way of both David San Miguel and his rare vision, and Gemini Adams who raised the bar and challenged me to get this right.

Eternal gratitude to Julie Bond Genovese, my Anam Cara, and in memory of my darling Syuta Gudemann (1906-2010) who never neglected to ask, "How's Mother?"

Finally, I thank Todd and Eliza for loving both Cecy and me with unending courage and humor.

THE FOG

I.

Painted Wings

Alone in her room,
She shifts and sorts
The mountains of paper that shape
The boundary of her world.

Each letter derails her better sense
And sends her seeking solace
In a talking head
On the sure, black box.

There was an owl once,
Perched and determined,
Outside the glass portal
Separating her from time.

Daily, he'd come,
Spectacular and wild,
Encouraging flight
From her papered nest.

One ardent morning,
Traversing a ledge of missives,
She peered through the pane
To find him gone.

Oil-based, now,
Grounded and mute,
He lives upon her wall.
Good company for the six o'clock news.

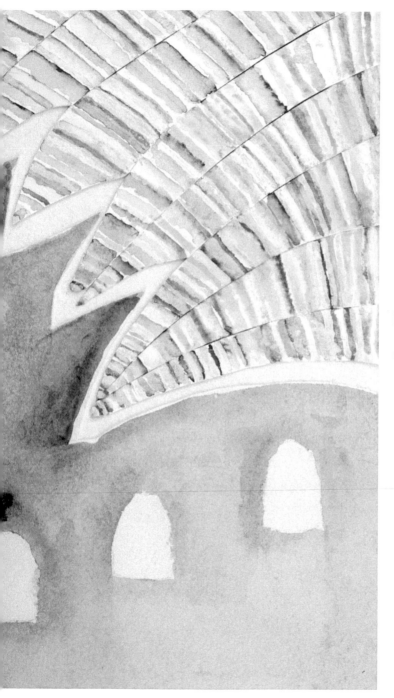

Susan Winn: Cecy's cousin-in-law. Watercolor and collage, Maine 2010.

3

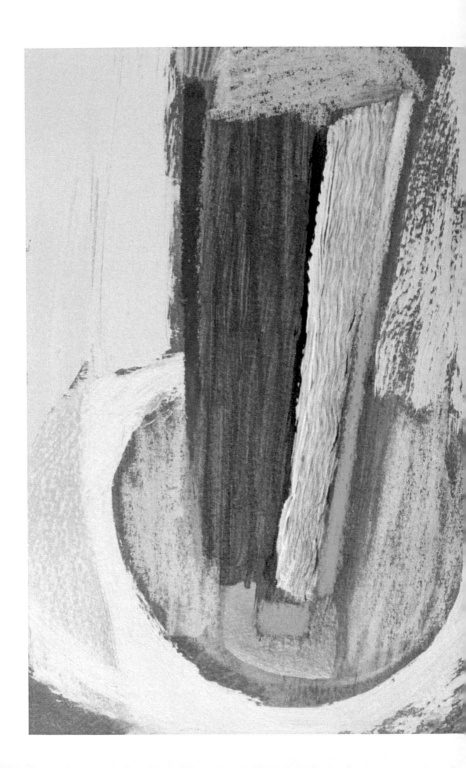

Measuring Up

A silhouette not as tall
Not as stately
Of slighter frame.

A temperament
Not as sharp
Not as Irish
Of subtler nature.

A wit
Not as quick
Not as wicked
Of hesitant word.

A pride
Not as glowing
Nor righteous
Of humbler grain.

A loss
No less poignant
Nor devastating
Of gargantuan proportion.

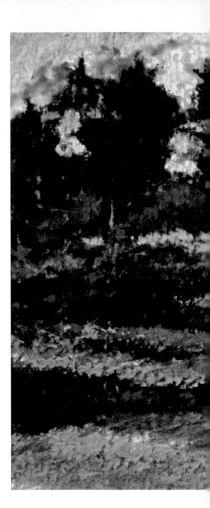

The Seagull

Like Nina, she wanted to be a seagull.
"No that's not it…"
She wanted to soar, unencumbered,
Sounding plaintive calls for peace.

She wanted to be a seagull.
To live and die
Flying high above the coast of Maine.
Black firs silhouetted against mackerel sky.

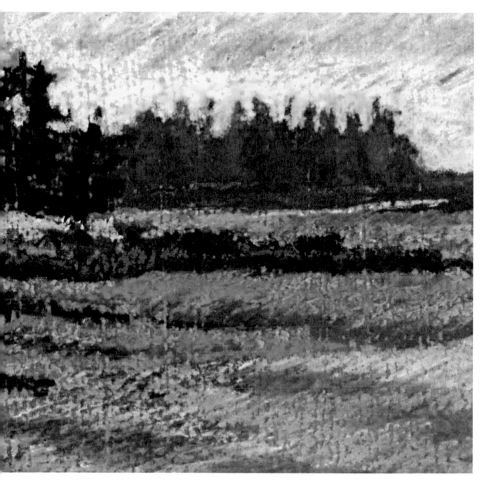

Tom Prescott: Cecy's son. Pastel on paper, Maine 2006.

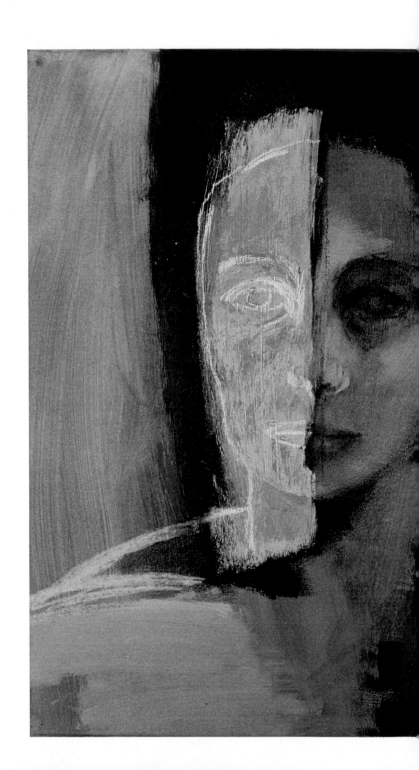

Mother's Lullaby

Anne Gresinger: Cecy's niece. Acrylic on paper, Maine 1993.

For a moment I saw you
Now specter, once stalwart
Sober voiced, sharp with wisdom
Focused clean near the ache.

You showed yourself briefly
Over steak spiked with history
I sensed you re-circuit
Those raw, well-worn days.

Dire sorrow plays harshly
On one fine of tuning
I watched you change stations
Ride wild toward the dawn.

Bone-white light sheds comfort
Lifts shadow, hides memory
Shines blithely down pathways
Impervious to pain.

II.

NOR'EASTER

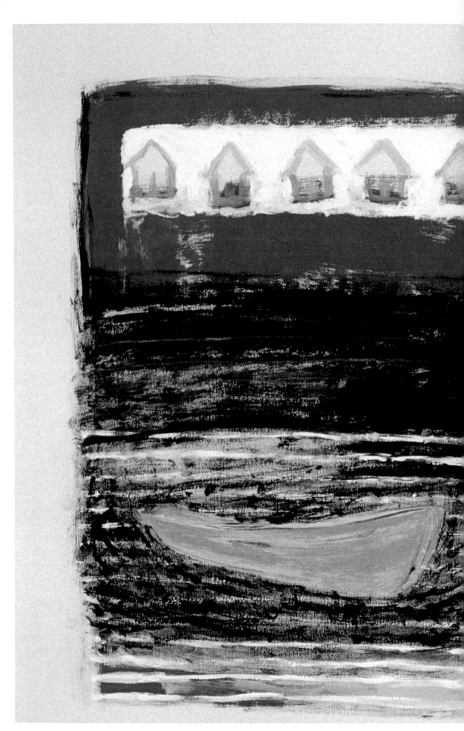

Proof

She disappears before me,
Silently slipping into a realm
In which I don't figure,
Quietly busying herself with
New vistas, devoid of reason.

If she cannot know me
Do I exist?
My history is erased systematically,
As each neuron misfires
And no longer seeks its intended connection.

As the night rain displaces
The dust of daily life,
So am I displaced,
Destined to build my own boat
And sail to higher ground.

Anne Gresinger: Cecy's niece. Acrylic on paper, Maine 1984.

Gone
New connections
Depth abandoned
Mama's missing
Gone in a blaze
Flattened by iron
Grayed like ash
Mama in stories
Pretend and pretend
Mama, oh Mama
Mama is dying

Gone

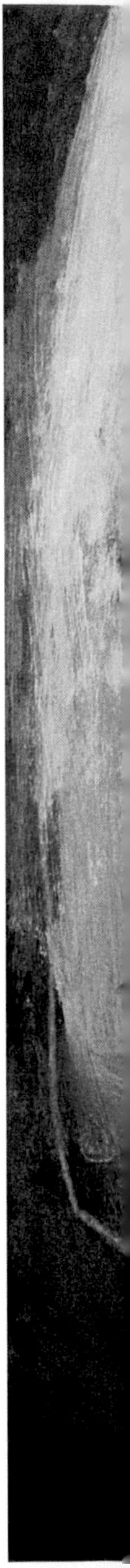

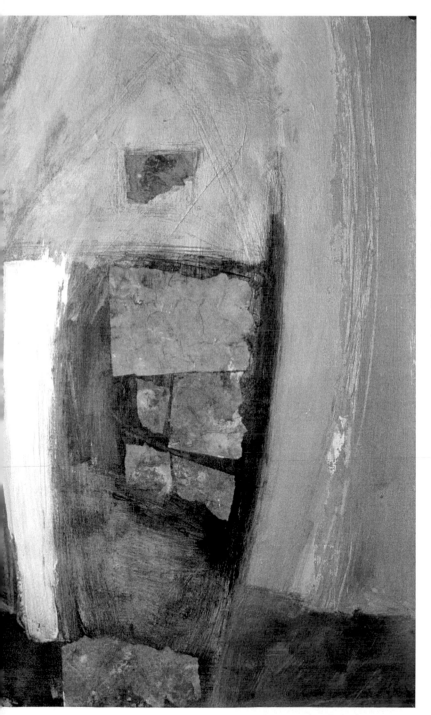

Anne Gresinger: Cecy's niece. Mixed media on paper, Maine 1986.

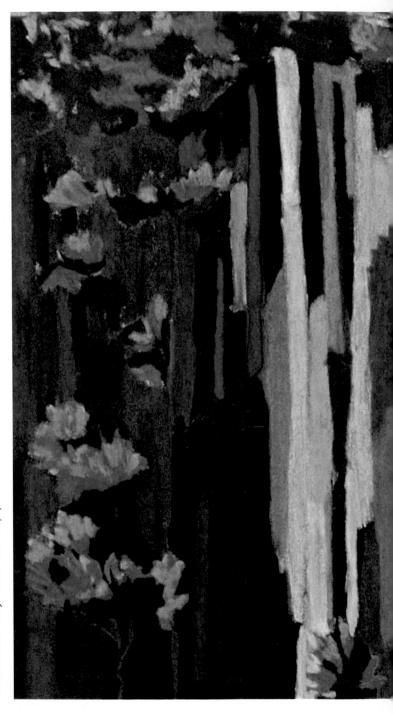

Tom Prescott: Cecy's son. Pastel on paper, Maine 2006.

The under-bricking,
The over arching,
The hand of doing,
Yes, handy
Doing.

Glamorous lady,
Witty
And sad.

Holding a world
Together
With rubber bands,
Paper clips,
And sealing wax.

Quick Hold

The screen door opens,
The night breeze flashes,
It flies up stairwells,
But you aren't there.

Asleep in mind,
My mind, my memory,
My Mother lies sleeping
In corners of time.

Mother

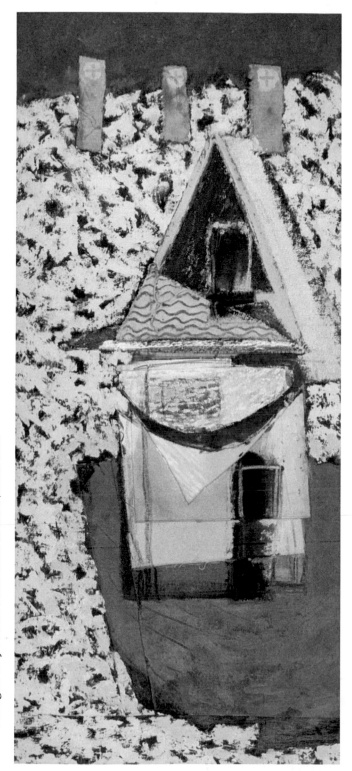

Anne Gresinger: Cecy's niece. Mixed media on canvas, Maine 1986.

III.

EBB TIDE

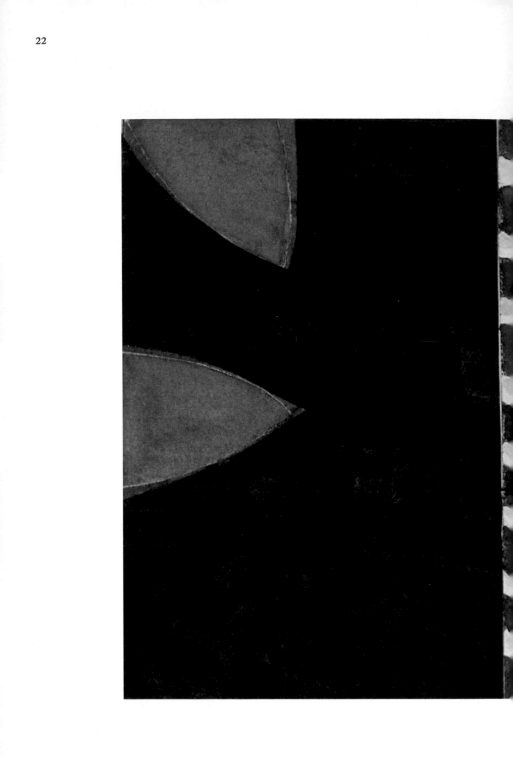

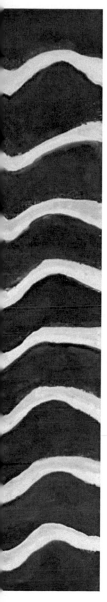

Susan Winn: Cecy's cousin-in-law. Watercolor and collage, Maine 2010.

Silent Sea

Bright eyes
Deepest blue
Dimmed milk-white
Searching, struggling
Floating backwards
To warmer waters
In desperate hope
Of light

Black ice
Fierce, intruding
Restructures sense

Bluest eyes
Brilliant blue
Empty

Tidal ebb
The sea
Is silent

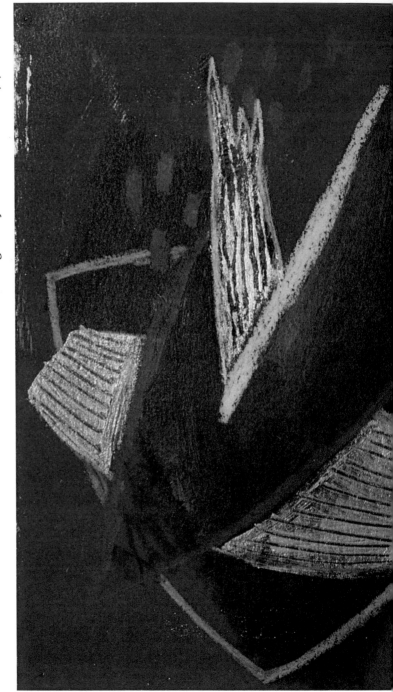

Anne Gresinger: **Cecy's niece.** Mixed media on paper, Maine 1992.

Unveiled

Gorgeous woman.
Song of grace
Of feature
Magnetizing force
Destructive to her path.

Beauty so tempting.
Triumph of wit
Troubling bait
For exploit
Deceit.

Threat to her.
Bounty to him.
Alone
Unsure
Romantic, yet weary.

In search of love
In a house of cards.

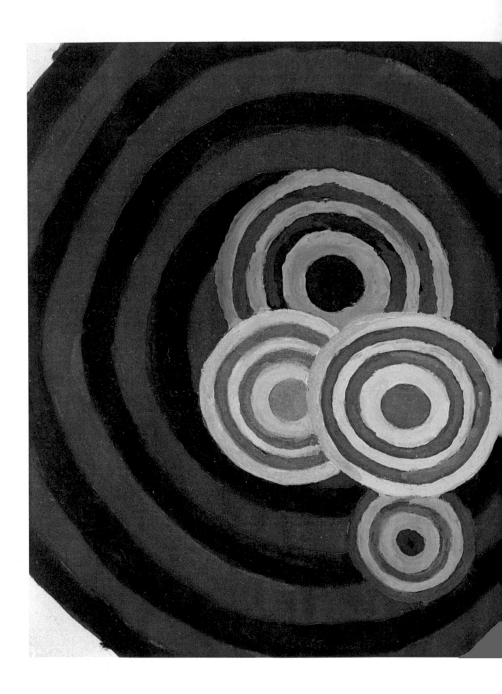

Mother, I'm tired.
I've tried to bury you,
Resurrect you, rediscover you.
I am in a magic disappearing booth
Waiting for the trick to end.

What kind of magician
Would allow me
To step out of the booth
Into a world
Devoid of you?

Vanishing

Home

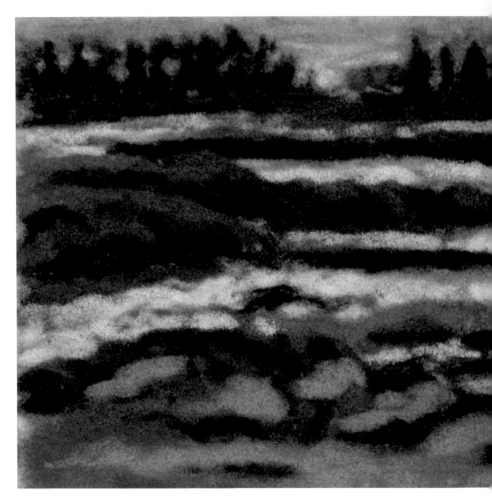

Tom Prescott: Cecy's son. Pastel on velour paper, Maine 2006.

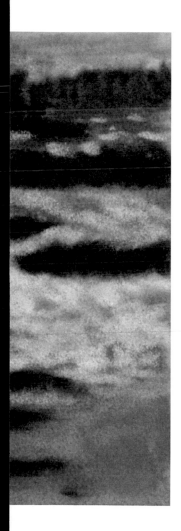

Barnacles shining on slippery rocks,
I step barefoot upon the weeds.
Tidal pools warm with bugs,
Walking their watery film.
Periwinkles, half emerged,
Looking to cling,
To ride out the waves.

Tweedy green rope
Caught between the shelves,
I see the tumble of water
Beneath me.

Cast me out
To the farthest bell.
Let me lie there
Quietly with the seals.
I want to heal
To it's rhythmic gong.

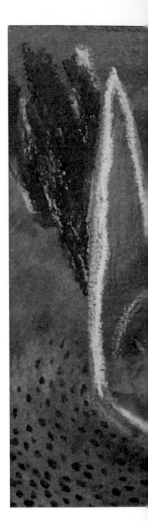

Beyond all organized thought,
In the presence of extreme dementia,
There exists an awareness of love.

A love that grounds one, however briefly,
A faint glow of better times
When humor reigned and language flowed.

There is desire on a moonless night
To spot a firefly,
To stumble through deafening blackness
To mark its winged flight.

For one brief second,
Hovering high above the grass, it burns,
A love stronger than forgetting
Shining in contempt of the dark.

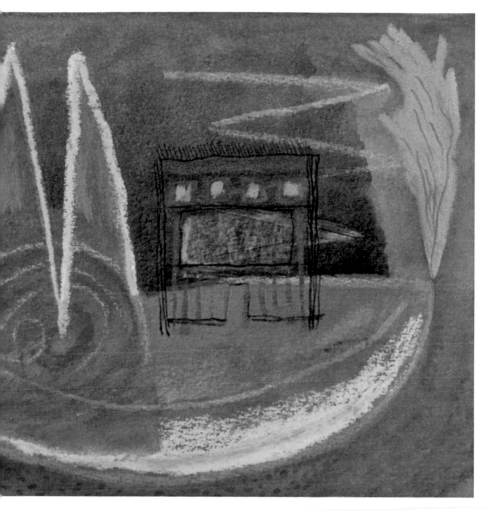

Anne Gresinger: Cecy's niece. Mixed media on paper, Maine 1992.

Firefly

IV.

MACKEREL SKY

Sexy and Cecy

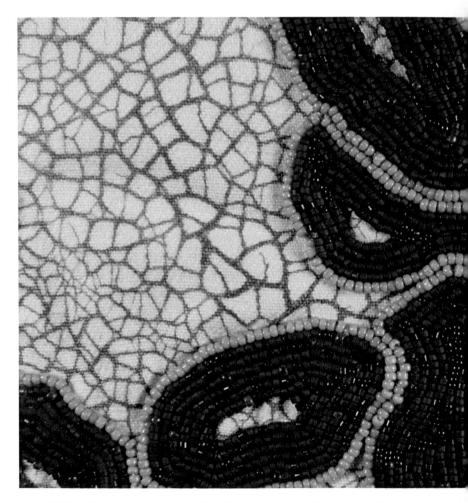

Susan Winn: Cecy's cousin-in-law. Glass beads on printed fabric, Maine 2006.

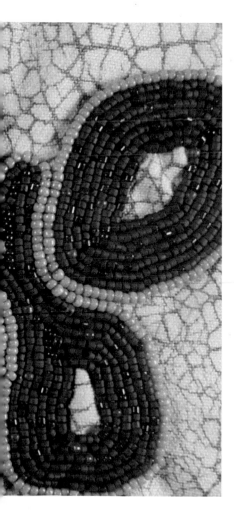

I remember. I do.
The men faltered.
You, straight and strong.
Beauty electric.

They followed,
Like so many salmon,
Flipping and climbing.

Afraid your bright eyes,
Might look away.

Sexy and Cecy,
Clean, tragic, delight.

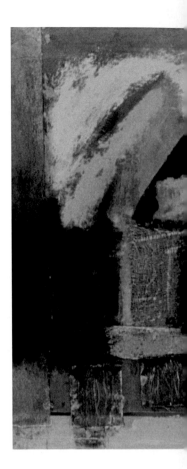

You made candles in Mateus bottles,
Sat in waist high reeds on Damariscove,
Wore your hair in braids.

The farm, where it all hangs out,
"Cecilia" playing on eight track,
Weaving your macrame belts.

Sperry top-siders for the boat.
Chamois shirt concealing
The history of your mother.

Party husband, madras shorts,
Weekend commuter dad.
Alone, you dreamed.

You learned to make fishing nets,
Funny wooden needle, tying knots,
To catch you when you fall.

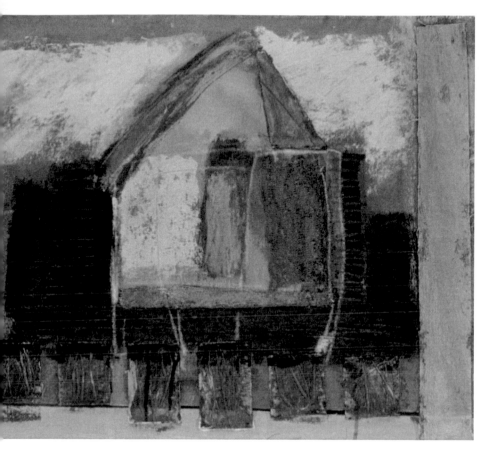

Anne Gresinger: Cecy's niece. Acrylic on canvas, Maine 1986.

Fishing Nets

V.

IN IRONS

I leap off the board
A perfect swan dive
Into an unsettled sea

Devoid of the old
Immersed in the new
Tired, unsure, alone

Flailing, rolling, heavy
Cloaked in a shawl of desperation
Wrestling the tide

Righteous, fogged, impatient
I beach myself
Brittle as a crab

Scuttling the slippery rocks
Barnacled and black with slime
Lousy with fear

Blind to the sun, the reeds, the blue
Numb to the winds
That could sail me back home

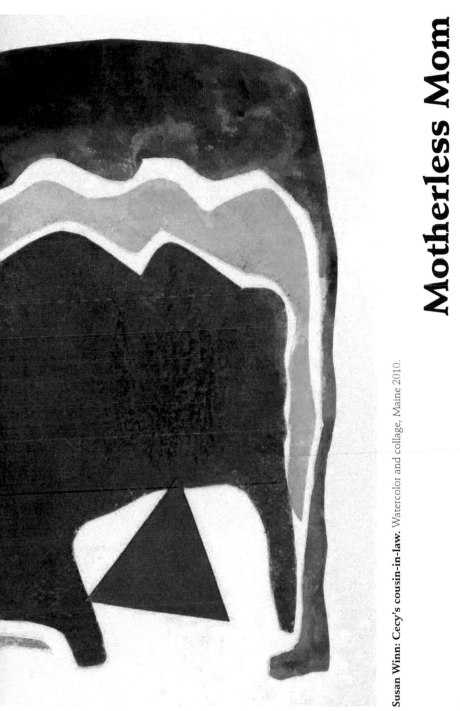

Motherless Mom

Susan Winn: Cecy's cousin-in-law. Watercolor and collage, Maine 2010.

Anne Gresinger: Cecy's niece. Mixed media on canvas, Maine 1986.

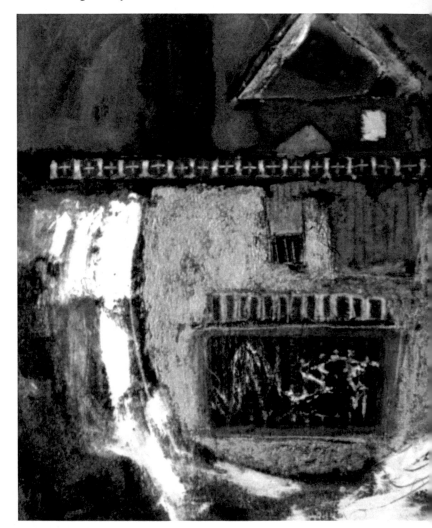

Bon Voyage

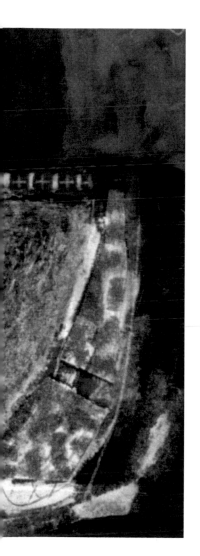

Sometimes it's better to loosen
the spring line
and let her
float away.

If the storm is that great,
why keep her tethered,
battering herself to pieces
at the dock?

Let her go.
Watch her float peacefully away
under a grey and turbulent sky.

A last grand sail into
whatever lies beyond.

A graceful exit from all things
measured and charted.

Beautiful ketch,
I release you.

VI.

FOLLOWING SEA

I could take you by the hand.
We could hop a moving train.
I could ride you on my handlebars
Far from this dreary lane.

I could flag a passing cab.
Tell the driver, "hurry…quick!"
I could start up an old outboard.
Give the engine one swift kick.

If I'd wings, I'd surely fly you.
I've a map. I'd find the way.
I'd careen you back in time with me
To somewhere sense still lay.

Just hold my waist. Don't let me go.
The fog will lift. You'll see once more.
I'll not quit you. It's getting cold.
I'll lead you straight to your front door.

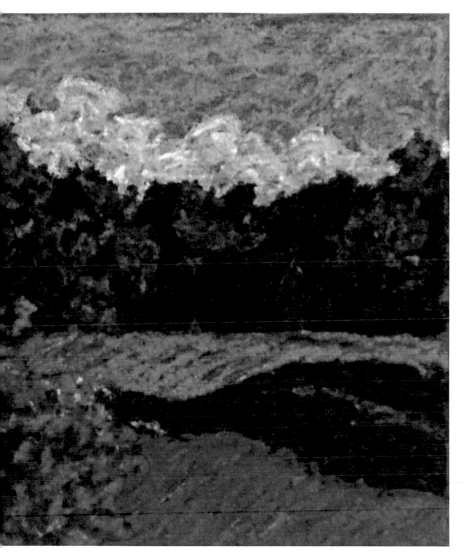

Tom Prescott: Cecy's son. Pastel on paper, Maine 2002.

"Let's Just Get Home,"
she said...

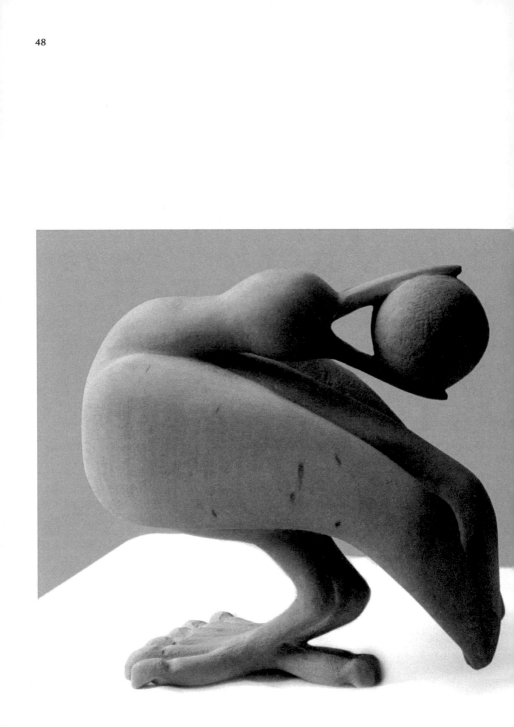

Rosanne MacPherson: Cecy's sister-in-law. Bass wood carving, Maine 2009.

Thoughtless as a peek into the fledglings' nest
A frantic ruffle of feather and bone
Tiny birds test half-baked wings
Falling to the earth

Mother gone in search of food
Returns to meticulously woven twigs
Her brood undone

A wild dance to recover, to regain
Sacrifice and vigilance in shambles
The phoenix searches her embers
A hope of burning life
Beneath the leaves

Fledglings

There is a level of vibration,
Voice to ear,
That surpasses all obstruction.

An echo of synapse and bone
That leaps the highest hurdle
Eviscerating canon.

A sonorous "yes"
To a life
That is quietly failing.

The sounding hum
Of a love
Too deep
To mute.

Hello

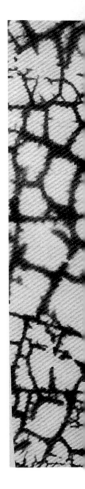

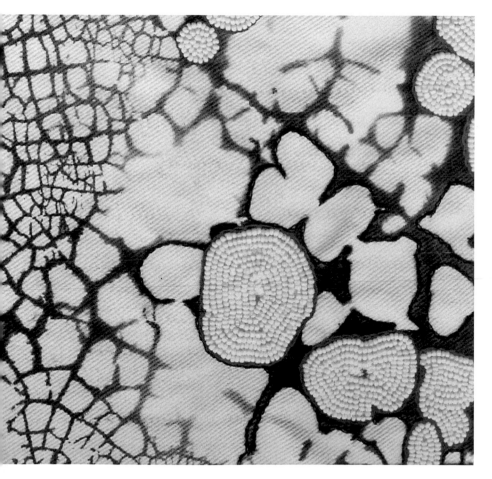

Susan Winn: Cecy's cousin-in-law. Glass beads on printed fabric, detail, Maine 2006.

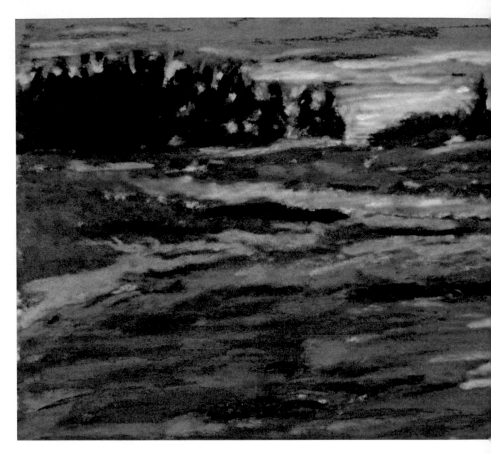

Tom Prescott: Cecy's son. Pastel on paper, Maine 2006.

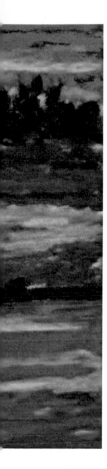

He sits, strong beside her
Bracing for the bumps.
Holding that hand
Once sticky with jam,
Then gloved and gay,
Now lined with years,
They rise.

Treading softly amongst moss and briar,
They stop briefly to check under the bed,
Shuffle the soft-shoe of a torch song,
Straighten a crooked tie.

Quayside, they pause,
Searching within, scanning the horizon.
He hands her passage,
The unmistakable grace
Of knowing and having been known.

Safe Passage

We stepped over, hand in hand, to the covered swing

Its round, plump form devoid of feather

Her long legs pushed with the memory of strength

Complete stillness, just the translucent form of hope

Brittle, bird-like bones lying against mine

A red spot beside us…perhaps the point of impact

We flew, singing to sturdier ground

Hidden in the corner above…the telltale twigs

Rocking to sleep, imprinted on my shoulder

Bounced from seat to burning sidewalk, it squats

A wish for that final, weighty flight

Finished in a valiant posture of success

Birds of a feather

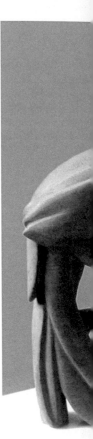

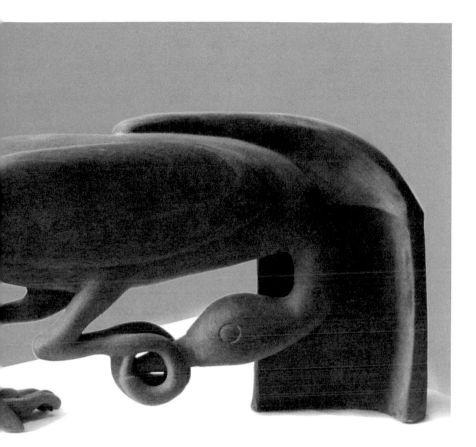

Rosanne MacPherson: Cecy's sister-in-law. Mahogany carving, Maine 2001.

Birds of a Feather

VII.

Red, Right, Returning

To seize is to hold,
To take hold of.
To squeeze sense from,
Or shake sense into?
To slyly awaken,
Or block what remains?

I seize your fingers,
Cold in mine,
Bony, anxious, searching.

I cannot hold you.
Derail your impulse
To find the latch
To the dusty tome
That housed your dreams.
Written in a child's hand,
That you might
Begin again.

Seizures

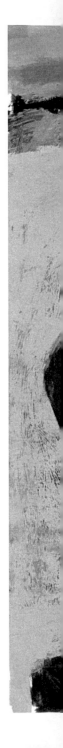

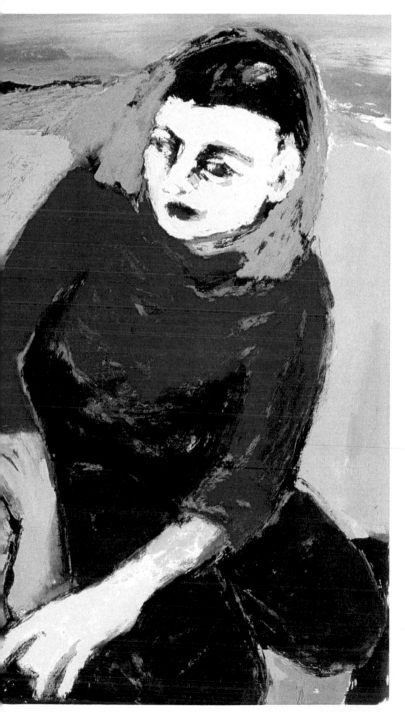

Anne Gresinger: Cecy's niece. Acrylic on paper, Maine 1990.

Irony Lost

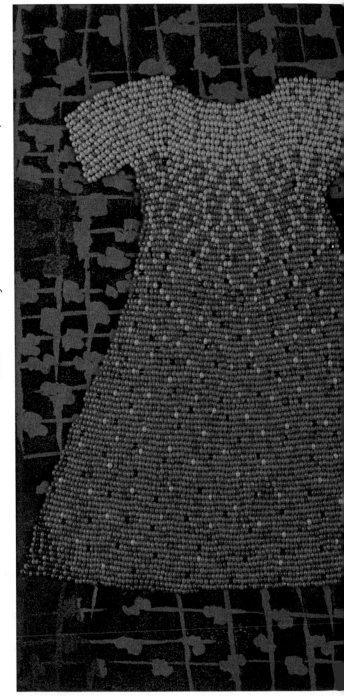

Susan Winn: Cecy's cousin-in-law. Glass beads on printed fabric, Maine 2006.

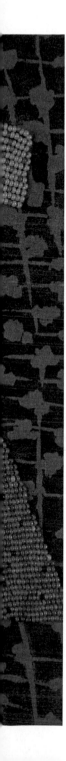

I crease your brow,
Cause you upset.
It's discourteous as hell, Mom,
And I'm sorry for it.

I'm not there anymore...
Not calling to tell you I'm leaving the party,
Not shocking you with my irreverence,
Not needing to, "do something with that hair."

I'm just not there for you, Mom.
You scrunch, you search, you poke my cheek
But you can't find me.
Some daughter, eh?

Not even so much as an ...
"Olly olly oxen free!"
Nothing.
Not a clue.

I suppose I won't be back, Mom.
Sorry for the confusion.
I'm gone, see.
You've forgotten.

Mirage

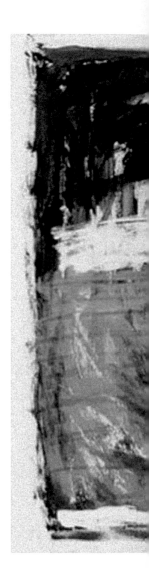

Drifting into the dock,
You extend a hand, pull me in,
Steady my dinghy as I disembark.

Carrying my oars,
You stumble on a root.
A fall, limbs all akimbo.

Fog, sudden as a sneeze.
Groping the air, I lunge for you,
Clawing the sodden moss.

The glint of an oarlock,
A flap of wings,
And you are gone.

Anne Gresinger: Cecy's niece. Acrylic on paper, Maine 1984.

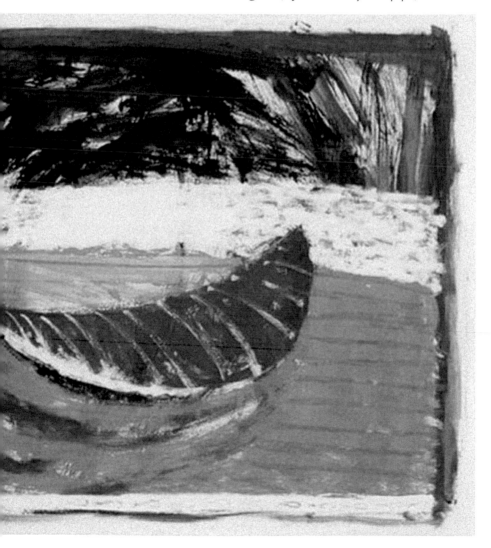

I wear a cape as I walk down the street,
A lovely large cape that goes down to my feet.
I fasten it carefully beneath my chin,
The wind is so furious and I am so thin.
Well, that is the story I'm willing to tell.
The truth is quite different. I'm not little Nell.

There's a hole here, you see, the size of a pie plate,
Beneath my left shoulder. Yes, it seems this is my fate.
The wind whistles through me in the key of plain C.
I've tried humming and singing and slapping my knee.
Nothing will stop this loud hullaballoo.
I think if you heard it you'd wear a cape too.

The hole can't be filled in, no matter the angle.
Mud is too heavy and yarn, just a tangle.
Been empty a while now, I can't say just when.
I've kicked out two sparrows, a mouse, and a wren.
This hole is my lot and I'm sure you'll agree,
The cape offers solace for kazoo playing me.

In Confidence

I'm open to any new options you hear of.
The quickest of fixes are ones I steer clear of.
The truth is, a part of me's out on vacation.
To see her again would be cause for elation.
I dream that she knows me and utters my name.
To achieve this small feat would end this whole game.

The hole would fill in. It would be a fine day.
I'd hang up my cape, try to dress a new way.
But for now, I'll keep whistling and searching the sky
For a sign that all's well, that there's no need to cry.
I'll walk, run, and stumble until I learn why
The tune that I'm playing can't fathom, "goodbye."

I Hear You

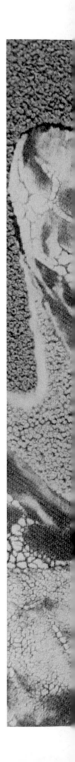

The voice conveys a gravity
So many icy
Crystalline stars
Wedged
Ever frozen
Into its tissue
Immune to heat
Mired in fortune

The inutterable
Spoken
On every breath
A gorgeous record
Of unfathomable depth
For all to hear

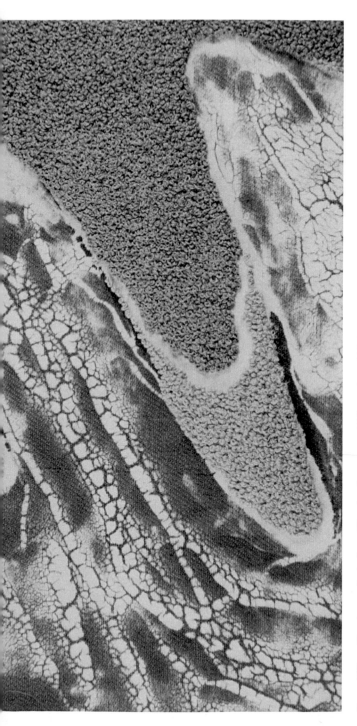

Susan Winn: Cecy's cousin-in-law. Glass beads on printed fabric, Maine 2006.

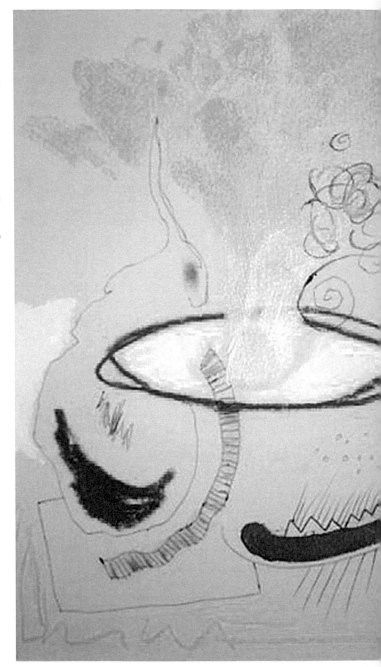

Anne Gresinger: Cecy's niece. Mixed media on paper, Maine 1994.

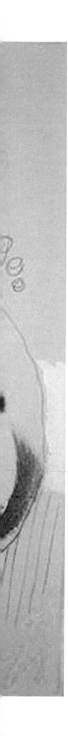

Stymied

i cannot
stop
you
falling
your
whirligig
yellow
window
dance

you wiggle
and
twirl
into
the earth
without
a
thought
of me

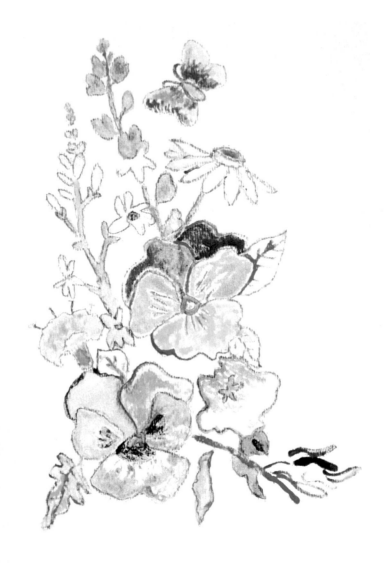

70

Cecy: assisted living. Colored pencil, Maine 2005.

Gather me
Like so many sticks
Scattered about the fire
One on top of the other
Layer me

Give me a roundness
A breadth
Afford me a space to fill
With vine, leaf, loam

I need to be an orchard
Vast and swaying
Laden with fruit
Not ash

Resolute

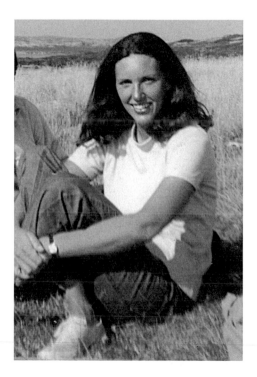

Cecy. Maine, 1970.

Your Contribution

A percentage of the proceeds from the sale of this book will be donated to the Alzheimer's Association, Maine Chapter. More than 37,000 Mainers are currently living with Alzheimer's disease, and nearly 150,000 friends and family members provide unpaid care for them.

The Alzheimer's Association, Maine Chapter, is the only statewide non-profit agency dedicated solely to those affected by memory disorders. Our comprehensive program of services is funded almost exclusively through the generosity of private donors and includes a 24/7 Helpline, care consultation, education and training for families and professionals, legislative advocacy, Safe Return, support groups, and more.

The mission of the Alzheimer's Association is to eliminate Alzheimer's disease through the advancement of research; to provide and enhance care and support for all affected; and to reduce the risk of dementia through the promotion of brain health. Our vision is a world without Alzheimer's.

For more information about the programs and services of the Alzheimer's Association, Maine Chapter, call 800-272-3900.

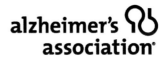

www.alz.org/maine

About the Author

Judy Prescott, born in Mountain Lakes, New Jersey, has spent the past twenty-five years working as a professional actress. Based in both New York City and Los Angeles, she has performed many roles on stage and screen. Her most recent work includes episodes of *True Blood*, *Grey's Anatomy*, *Cold Case*, *Bones*, and the films *Islander* and *Hit and Runway*.

Judy started writing poems as a child in order to better understand the world around her. She began reading her poetry publicly fifteen years ago in Los Angeles where she currently lives with her husband and daughter.

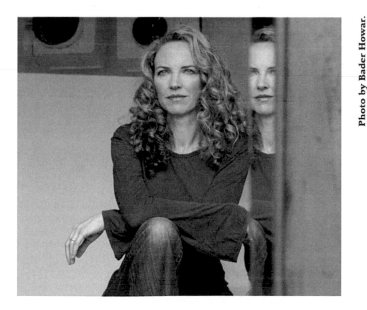

About the Type

F. H. Ernst Schneidler designed Schneidler Old Style in 1936. Stempel Schneidler is based on the typefaces of Venetian printers from the late fifteenth century and possess their grace, beauty, and classical proportions. One of Stempel Schneidler's most recognizable features is it's rare question mark. An editorial decision was made to use Garamond for all of the question marks in this book.